I10701638

SAFETY TIPS THAT CAN SAVE YOUR BUTT!

Lifesaving tips from a firefighter/paramedic

SAFETY TIPS THAT CAN SAVE YOUR BUTT!

Martin Lesperance

Safety Health Publishing Inc.

Martin Lesperance "Safety Tips that can save your butt!"

Copyright © 2002 Martin Lesperance

Published by Safety Health Publishing Inc.
Calgary, Alberta, Canada. 1-888-278-8964

Lesperance, Martin, 1953-
Safety Tips That Can Save Your Butt
ISBN: 0-9730587-0-6
1. Accidents — Prevention. I. Title.
HV675.L47 2002   363.1   C2002-910616-8

Editor and layout: Dave Lowery
Illustrations: Jacqueline Dube
Cover design: Kathi Dunn

DISCLAIMER
The author and publisher have checked with sources believed to be reliable in a conscientious effort to provide information that is complete and congruent with acceptable standards at the time of publication. However, the dynamic nature of this information leads to anticipate future changes and updates. Therefore, readers are encouraged to confer with other reliable sources to ensure that they will receive complete, accurate and current information.

Printed in Canada

INTRODUCTION

Since I've been working as a firefighter/paramedic for around twenty years, I've managed to pick up a lot of stories. Most firefighters like to tell them so when I speak at safety conferences and meetings I'm often told that the attendees loved my stories. Since I'm a pretty good story teller I've had people come up to me six months later and tell me they still remembered certain ones and the safety point I made. If people remembered the story, they remembered the message. Because people learn from stories, I've collected some interesting ones in this book. Each story refers to a safety message and each chapter has a different message with some solid advice and information.

The beginning of the book talks about the cost of injuries and how you, your family and your employer will be affected if you're injured. Some of these stories are not happy, but injuries are not happy events.

I also talk about the misuse of the word "accident" and how we have to look at the word in a different light. Statistics are covered in a different way than you're used to.

Throughout the book will be some pretty amazing stories. True stories. I was there for many of them.

This book is meant to be entertaining but more importantly, it is meant to help you remember some safety tips. It is also meant to help you learn from other people's mistakes. Many people who have been injured hope that other people can learn from their mistakes.

Safety isn't a joke; it's one of the most important things you can practice for you and your family. Safety isn't a joke . . . but it can be fun.

— Martin Lesperance 2002

Table of Contents

Chapter

1

WEAR CLEAN UNDERWEAR; YOU NEVER KNOW WHEN YOU'LL BE IN AN ACCIDENT!

For years, your mother has been telling you to wear clean underwear because you never know when you're going to be in an "accident." I didn't put much thought into that until I started working as a paramedic. Then momma's advice started to make sense.

Contrary to popular belief, few cowboys died in gunfights. Most were killed from horse related injuries. Many died from drowning while crossing rivers during trail drives. Another big killer was prostate cancer.

If you're involved in an "accident" and you're seriously injured, here's what is going to happen. The ambulance will pull up and the paramedics are going to pull out some big scissors to cut off your clothes. We do this to look for further injuries before we move you. Then we'll treat the injuries, place you on the stretcher and take you to the hospital. In the hospital, we'll tell the hospital staff what happened and where you're injured. Then we'll leave to clean up our ambulance and do the paper work.

As we're cleaning up the ambulance, my partner and I will talk. We won't talk about how good an employee, hockey player or parent you are. What we'll talk about (and I realize this is totally unfair but who said life is fair) is what kind of a person you are by the condition of your underwear. Since this is probably the first time we have met you, we don't have a lot to go on but what we see in front of us. First impressions do count!

We do have a rating system. It goes from one to five. One means mom would have been really proud of you while five means . . . well it means you must have been really, really scared.

So now you know the reason why mothers across the continent have been telling their children to wear clean underwear.

2

THE RIPPLE EFFECT OF AN INJURY

When most of us take a risk, whether it's running a yellow light in your vehicle or standing on the "this is not a step" warning on a step ladder, we rarely think about the consequences of our actions. The last thing we think about is "what will happen if things go wrong?" If I get hurt, how will I be affected and who else will be affected? When was the last time you had these thoughts before you took a risk?

The following is a story about a guy who never dreamed things would end up like they did.

We were told to respond to a house where the 9-1-1 dispatcher said two young children were screaming hysterically on the front yard. As we pulled up we recognized the house. About eight months earlier, the man who lived there had fallen off a roof and fractured his pelvis, thighbone, knee and some vertebrae in his back. They were very serious fractures. This man, who was once very active and participated in running, hockey and fishing, suddenly became bed ridden.

He didn't handle this situation very well and became addicted to the painkillers he was taking. He also started to drink heavily. He became very withdrawn because he didn't want his friends to see him in this condition. He ignored his wife's pleas for him to get help and thought he could handle his problem by himself. Finally she couldn't take it any longer so she packed up, took the kids and left. His substance abuse and anger increased until one afternoon he took his walker and shuffled across the living room down the hallway into the bathroom. He stepped into the bathtub, closed the shower curtain, placed the end of the barrel of the shotgun he was carrying in his mouth and pulled the trigger.

This was the day his kids decided to pay daddy a visit. They were the ones who found him.

This example is extreme, but situations like this do happen. Below are some ways a person can be affected after a serious injury occurs whether it happens on or off the job.

- Injuries cause pain and suffering to the injured person.
- Injuries will add stress to the injured person and to the people close to them.
- Financial difficulties may result.
- Lowered self-esteem, a sense of worthlessness and withdrawal from society are possible.

A plane blew up at 33,330 feet over Czechoslovakia. One of the flight attendants survived the fall. She was pronounced dead at the hospital but things changed. She was in a coma for 27 days. Sixteen months later she was discharged from the hospital.

An injury also affects your employer no matter where it happens

Benefit plans are expensive privileges that are there when you need them. When a worker is injured, either on or off the job, a tremendous ripple effect occurs. The following are just a few of the added costs.

- The worker has to be replaced, sometimes at overtime wages.
- Replacement workers may have to be trained causing lost productivity.
- Managers have to devote more time to the training of the replacement worker.
- Administration costs rise.
- When an employee is off work for an extended period, it is often difficult for them to return to work.
- Disability insurance or workers' compensation rates rise.
- Morale problems — when someone is seriously injured or killed, everyone who was close to that person is affected.

As you can see, there are many hidden costs involved. This added expense makes it more difficult for an employer to compete in the global market. As a result, everyone's job security could be affected.

We should all try to reduce injuries whether we are at home, work or play. If we can do this, it's a win-win situation for everyone involved. Your employer reduces payout for needless injuries but more importantly, you live a longer, happier life.

DON'T BECOME A VICTIM YOURSELF

A lady had a flat tire on a busy highway. She pulled over on to the shoulder and was attempting to change the flat. A man noticed her plight and pulled his vehicle over to offer assistance. As he attempted to help her he was struck by another vehicle and was killed instantly.

At a gas plant a man was overcome by hydrogen sulfide (a very poisonous gas) doing a procedure he had done many times before. A co-worker saw him lying unconscious and immediately ran to help him. He was also overcome. Another worker ran to help his friends. He, too, was overcome. Other workers saw this and took the appropriate emergency procedures including putting on their self contained breathing apparatus. They pulled the men to safety. Unfortunately it was too late for two of them. They died.

The most important part of any rescue is the safety of the rescuers. I can not stress this enough. If you go to help someone and become a victim yourself, you are not only useless to the person who needs the help, you complicate matters.You have to be rescued also.

When an emergency situation occurs it is very easy for tunnel vision to occur. Tunnel vision is what happens when you see a situation and all your attention focuses on that situation. You become oblivious to your surroundings including your own safety. This kills many people every year and it can happen very easily.

If you ever come across an emergency such as a house fire, motor vehicle collision, shooting or anything else you can imagine, before you attempt to help you must stop, take a good look around, look for further danger that may be obvious or not, assess the situation and then decide how you are going to act.

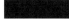

In some cases the best thing you can do is run away. Protect yourself. Attempting to help a person when it's unsafe to do so can get you killed. It may be a difficult decision, but it is the right decision.

A paramedic attended a small plane crash. The pilot was dead and the passenger had a serious head injury. Aviation fuel was everywhere. Without waiting for the fire truck to arrive to handle the possible fire, he crawled into the plane and dragged the injured person out. The passenger died shortly after.

This paramedic was suspended from work for putting himself in such danger. He was then nominated for a medal of bravery.

There is a very fine line between being a hero and a person who made a horrible error in judgment. In this situation, the difference between a hero and a stupid person was a spark.

Don't become a victim yourself!

A British woman was suffering from chronic fatigue. She decided to fix herself so she took a drill and, in front of a mirror and video camera, drilled a two-centimeter hole in her skull. She not only survived but said she felt much better after doing it. I wouldn't recommend any of my readers, or anyone else, try this.

4

NEVER BE AFRAID TO CALL AN AMBULANCE

Call me an ambulance . . . okay, you're an ambulance! While providing advanced life support, paramedics can occassionally encounter miscommunication at scenes, possibly due to the extrememly high pressure people experience during an emergency.

One young lady epitomized this following her father's cardiac arrest at a gas station.

After arriving to find the unfortunate man pulseless and not breathing, the crew began treatment and at the same time, asked the gathered crowd if anyone knew CPR, hoping for some assistance until fire or ambulance backup arrived.

Fearing her father to be without help, the young lady understandingly screamed, "You don't know CPR?!" (D.L.)

Hemorrhoids are a bummer, but they rarely kill

Most people have probably had a case or two of hemorrhoids while others may be cursed with them on a regular basis. They are not a lot of fun but I wouldn't really call them an emergency. Others would.

We responded to a house where the caller said he needed help. On arrival we saw a man sitting at the kitchen table smoking a cigarette and drinking a beer. It was obvious he wasn't on his first beer of the evening. He said his hemorrhoids were bothering him and he wanted a ride to the hospital. Because his condition wasn't an emergency we told him the ride would cost him about $120.00. (1982 prices.) He let out a scream and started laughing hysterically and said ,"I don't have to pay for this, you guys have to because I'm on social assistance." He continued laughing and slapping his thigh. His laugh was so contagious before you knew it we were laughing also.

Normally you are taught to try to visualize and physically examine the injured part, and since we didn't have a student we could have fun with, (we would have told the student "you gotta try to examine the 'rhoids") we just decided to give 'rhoid sufferer a ride to the hospital. Maybe his hemorrhoids were really bad and in that case I might have truly felt sorry for him. Maybe they were painful and bleeding but I don't know for sure. I didn't take a close look!

A very tough, not to mention, polite man.

In 1997 a Turkish farmer had a really bad toothache. The pain was so bad he told his friends he was going to blow the tooth out with a pistol. The bullet went through his head killing him instantly.

My partner and I were hanging around the emergency department waiting for a call. The waiting room was busy when a guy about 50 years of age walked in and asked to see a doctor. He was asked if his problem was serious and he said it wasn't. He was told to sit down until his name was called. I noticed he started to look a bit pale while sitting in the waiting room so I walked over and asked if he was okay. He looked at me and said "yes but my gut hurts." I asked him if he had injured it or if the pain came on by itself as many medical emergencies do. I remember his reply as he looked at me. "I've been shot." Being a bit surprised at his reply I asked how it happened? "While shooting a buffalo," he said. Maybe he had lost a lot of blood and wasn't thinking clearly so I asked him to explain. He worked for a small custom meat packing plant and a bullet had ricocheted off the skull of the, now, deceased buffalo and hit him in the gut. He was telling the truth. This was one very polite, not to mention, tough, man.

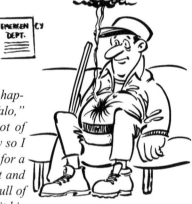

These are two extremes. One person calls an ambulance when it wasn't needed; the other gentleman needed one and didn't call. You should never hesitate or be afraid to call an ambulance if you need one.

Activating emergency medical services

If you or someone else needs help, never be afraid to call an ambulance, fire or police department. If you do need to make that call, here are a few tips to remember.

When someone needs an ambulance, police or fire department, they may be in a very serious situation or may have just witnessed a horrible scene. The anxiety level for everyone involved can go through the roof. Mistakes can be made when the caller is overly anxious. People can get so worked up in an emergency they can't even remember their own name. Seriously!

Here are a few things you should know and expect when you access 9-1-1 or the emergency number in your area.

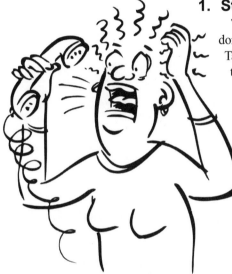

1. Stay Calm

This is easier said than done but it's very important. Take a deep breath and try to slow down your thinking. Try to stay calm. The person who is taking your call for help has done this before and will help you through the emergency. (Hopefully, it's not their first day on the job!)

2. Not all areas have 9-1-1

While most areas in North America use 9-1-1 as the emergency telephone number, there are areas that don't. Many rural areas are not set up for 9-1-1 so it's very important to know the telephone numbers for the fire, ambulance and police departments for your particular area. Keep them posted by the telephone. You could have people visiting and you're the one who needs the ambulance. Your visitors will need to know what emergency number to call.

3. Know your address. (This isn't as silly as it sounds.)

Most people know where they live especially in cities and towns where there are street addresses you can see (or should be able to see). Hopefully your house numbers aren't blocked by trees or vegetation and are visible from the street. Many people who live in apartment blocks or condomini-

An 82-year-old man died when his wife ran over him in the driveway. He had fallen and could not get up. He told his wife to drag him to the house with the car. She tied an extension cord to his belt but the belt broke. She then tied it to his ankle but it slipped off. The man then asked his wife to back the car up so he could reattach it. She got the brake mixed up with the gas and ran over him.

ums may not know the proper address for their complex. This becomes very important for the emergency people to help you. Know where you live.

Rural areas can be a big problem. A high percentage of people do not know the legal address of their farm or acreage. I've been called to respond to a farm where the caller gave the location and directions in a manner that were totally useless. The directions went something like this:

"Go two miles down the Old Mill Road. (It hadn't been called that for the past 10 years.)
Turn left at Wilson's house (I didn't know who the heck Wilson was) and go for about three miles or so till you see the granary. Turn right and we are the third purple house on the right. (Try looking for a purple house that is forty yards off the road at two o'clock in the morning during a rainstorm!) Good luck! Then they wonder what took us so long!

Emergency workers are not mind readers. Some of us may not even be very bright. We have to know the proper address to find it on the map. It's unlikely the paramedics responding to your area grew up near you. We may be city folk who have just moved to your area.

4. Give the Nature of the Call

It's important for the emergency personnel to know what kind of emergency they are responding to.

Once we responded to a man who, the caller said, was having chest pain. True heart attacks are sometimes encountered when the dispatcher sends emergency crews to a chest pain complaint. When we arrived to treat this gentleman, much to our amazement, we found the patient had been shot in the chest. We believed him when he said his chest was hurting but this was a surprise and it certainly changed our response and treatment. You become very nervous when someone has been shot and the police aren't there. The police have guns . . . we don't.

Also keep in mind, when making the call, that different agencies may have to be notified. If power lines are down, the power company has to be notified. If the road is icy at a motor vehicle crash, a sanding truck may be in order. If people are trapped, a rescue vehicle has to be sent. Let the person who is taking your call know what is going on so they can send the appropriate agencies.

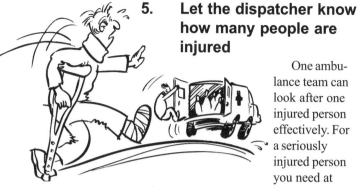

5. Let the dispatcher know how many people are injured

One ambulance team can look after one injured person effectively. For a seriously injured person you need at least two people to treat the patient and another to drive the ambulance. It can get very hectic at times. I'm sure most paramedics have had to treat several patients at one time or another. This is not a good situation which we try to avoid if possible. Let the dispatcher know how many people are injured so they can make the decision about how many ambulances to respond.

6. Give the telephone number you are calling from

Just in case the dispatcher has to get back to you, it's important for them to have your phone number.

7. Don't hang up first

Remember that the dispatcher is trained to take your call. It may seem like they are asking too many questions, and some may even sound silly at the time, but the questions are important. What usually happens is they will respond the ambulance while still talking to you. The ambulance is on the way but the questioning still continues. Once the dispatcher is satisfied they have enough information, they will relay the information to the emergency vehicles that are enroute to help. In some situations they may try to keep you on the phone until the help arrives to give you instructions such as how to perform CPR, control bleeding, assist in child birth and a plethora of other medical emergencies.

Some progressive emergency centres have a system in place called Medical Priority Dispatch (MPD). MPD was developed in the late seventies by Dr. Jeff Clawson, a practicing emergency physician in Salt Lake City, when he realized that dispatch was a weak link in the overall chain of survival. Dispatchers were considered as clerks, underestimated and

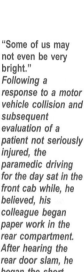

"Some of us may not even be very bright." *Following a response to a motor vehicle collision and subsequent evaluation of a patient not seriously injured, the paramedic driving for the day sat in the front cab while, he believed, his colleague began paper work in the rear compartment. After hearing the rear door slam, he began the short drive to the hospital. A few moments later, the paramedic noticed a small car pull up beside him at a traffic light and looked in the passenger seat. Sitting there was his partner, with a vehicle door handle still clutched in his hand — a souvenir from his desperate lunge at the departing ambulance's rear door. (D.L.)*

A 36-year-old man was golfing with his friends. Having a bad day and being extremely frustrated, he swung his club at a tree. The club broke and a piece of the shaft was propelled into his neck. He bled to death before reaching the hospital.

underutilized and he quickly determined this position needed protocols to be more effective. So he developed a card system where emergency medical dispatchers (EMD's) asked 9-1-1 callers key questions which led to appropriate responses by emergency agencies. But perhaps of more importance was that dispatchers now gave pre-arrival instructions to callers, a previously unheard of act, and eventually provided detailed instructions to help people through choking, childbirth, CPR and many other emergencies encountered. Callers in a community with EMD will be asked four key questions which will be:

1. Address, including phone number
2. A brief description of the problem
3. Is the patient conscious
4. Is the patient breathing.

Based on those four simple questions, the dispatcher will immediately send emergency agencies, especially if the answer to the third and fourth question is "no." It is critically important to stay on the phone with the EMD as they will then be able to read instructions from a card system to the caller on how to handle the emergency.

8. Don't make a call to 9-1-1 from a burning house!

If there is a fire in your home, get yourself and everyone out as safely and as quickly as you possibly can. Make the call for help from a neighbor's house or from a cell phone.

Once you're out of the house . . . don't go back in!

These are just a few tips to help you make an emergency call. Most local fire departments and ambulance services have information that may be specific in your area so check with them.

And this may seem obvious but it's important to emphasize that the emergency number to call is nine - one - one not nine - eleven. There are documented cases where people have delayed getting help because they were looking for the number eleven on the telephone key pad!

5

PAY ATTENTION TO WARNING SIGNS

I was speaking to a group of safety professionals at a conference and, since it was early December, talked about the number of people injured every year after they had fallen from stepladders while putting up their outside Christmas lights. After my talk, two safety professionals came up and quietly told me how they both had become injured in the same way. One of them admitted he was actually standing on the THIS IS NOT A STEP warning (how many times have you done this?), lost his balance and fell knocking himself unconscious. He would have frozen to death if the neighbor's child hadn't gone home and asked his mother why Mr. Smith was sleeping on the sidewalk. The second safety professional shattered his knee and was off work for four months.

Warning signs are there for a reason. Lawnmowers have warning signs telling people to keep their hands and feet away from underneath a running lawnmower. But every year, dozens and dozens of intelligent people will take a perfectly good hand and put it under a running lawnmower to grab something as valuable as an old stick or wet clump of grass.

Sometimes people will use lawnmowers for purposes they weren't designed; such as hedge trimmers. In theory, it may make sense to some. You get a willing helper to grab the other side of the running lawnmower, pick it up and carry it along the hedge but be very careful not to run (after all you could trip and hurt yourself). The scary part about this is people have actually done this. You have to wonder, what is going through their heads when they come up with an idea like this.

A man was staying at his mother's house while attending his father's funeral. While cleaning up the kitchen he tripped and fell onto the open door of the dishwasher. Two sharp utensils stabbed him. He died shortly after.

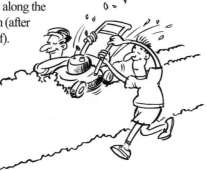

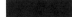

In Thunder Bay, Ontario, during 1998, eleven people came into city hospital emergency departments with serious hand injuries. The emergency physicians were wondering what the heck was going on but then realized it was the first heavy snowfall of the year and all the injuries were caused by snow blowers. So once again, seemingly intelligent people ignored the warning stickers and took a perfectly good hand and shoved it into a running snow blower to unplug the snow.

A 33-year-old man walked to the store to buy some bread and milk. On the way his buddy asked him in for a drink. After a few drinks he attempted to swallow his friends three-foot long sword. This was his first attempt at such a thing and he ended up cutting his throat and collapsing a lung. His wife, who was very understanding, said, "I love this man with all my heart but boy, what a jerk."

One person was finishing his basement using glue to lay the tiles on the concrete floor. On the glue container was a warning not to use the product near open flame. Unfortunately he did not realize that the pilot light on his water tank was an open flame and was quite close. When the fumes reached the pilot light they exploded. He received first and second degree burns to 25 percent of his body but was lucky! His injuries could have been more serious. Unfortunately, the resulting explosion and fire damaged his home extensively.

Warning signs are there for a reason.

We see warning signs wherever we go: stop signs warn us to stop, takeout coffee cups warn us the coffee is hot, gasoline containers warn us that gasoline is flammable and every electrical device known to man warns us we could be electrocuted if not used properly. (My photocopier even has a warning telling me I should unplug it when not in use . . . a fire may result if left plugged in!) I think many of the warnings are to cover the manufacturers' butts in case someone sues. But I realize most warnings are there for a good reason.

If you see warning labels on chemical containers, machinery, tools, or any recreational piece of equipment, pay attention to it. Remember they are there for a reason because people just as intelligent as you have been injured doing exactly what you plan on doing with that chemical or piece of equipment.

I once ignored a warning sign and, worse than that, I ignored a very smart local boy's advice.

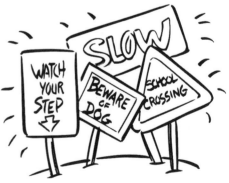

I was white water kayaking in Costa Rica for six weeks. One day I planned to go for a swim in the ocean. One of the local boys, who was about twelve years old, advised me in his broken English, that this part of the beach was "muy peligroso" (very dangerous) because of the riptide. Right behind him was a sign in Spanish and English warning of the riptide. But growing up in Winnipeg, and not spending any time around the ocean, I figured I probably knew more about oceans than this twelve-year-old kid because I was older and the warning sign was for people who didn't know how to swim well. When the kid left, I ran into the water but it wasn't long before I realized I was in trouble. The riptide was sucking me out to Africa and the shore was getting farther and farther away. Swimming against the current was useless because the current was stronger than me. At this point I was very concerned and crying for momma. I wondered why I didn't listen to that kid or pay attention to the warning sign. Remembering what the sign said to do if caught in a riptide, I swam parallel to the beach for approximately one hundred yards and then swam into the shore. My little swim ended up becoming a forty-five minute scare. This event could have been avoided if I listened to the boy and paid attention to the warning sign.

Pay attention to warning signs.

Chapter

6

MISUSE OF THE WORD ACCIDENT

There was a horrible car crash in Ontario, Canada, where five teenagers died. The next day, on national television, reporters interviewed one of the teenagers' friend who said she knew all of the people involved. What she said scared me as she looked into the camera."It was a horrible thing that happened – but it was an accident; it was just one of those things." This girls statement concerned me because it almost seemed to justify the crash and attempted to soften the impact.

I thought about some of the "accidents" I've attended in the past and especially about two guys snowmobiling after a few drinks I treated. They collided with each other and one died. It was an accident, it was just one of those things.

Then I thought about the grandfather taking his 10-year-old grandson hunting for the first time. As he stepped over a barbed-wire fence, his rifle discharged into the chest of his grandson killing him. It was an accident, it was just one of those things.

Then there was a three-year-old boy who lived in a fourth floor apartment. He was pushing on a screen and screens aren't designed to keep three-year-old boys in. He broke through and fell to his death but it was an accident, it was just one of those things.

On April 28, 1999 in Taber, Alberta, Canada, a high school student walked into the high school carrying a high-powered rifle and shot two students killing one of them. This made front-page news in every newspaper in North America. But the same day that student walked into the school and shot those students, an 18-month-old boy died when his father backed over him in the family driveway.

The same day that student walked into the school and shot those students, a five-year-old boy drowned in a dugout on the farm where he lived. You probably didn't hear or read about these deaths. They didn't make front-page news and were small write-ups on page eight of the local newspaper because, after all, these were "accidents." They were just one of those things.

An accident is not just one of those things.
Accidents are predictable and preventable events.
And they don't have to happen.

7

INJURIES THAT APPEAR MINOR, CAN SOMETIMES KILL

In some situations people can sustain potentially fatal injuries and survive. In some cases (thankfully not too often) people have been injured, taken to the hospital, examined, then sent home because their injuries did not appear to be serious. At home, they later died of their injuries as no medical system is foolproof. To complicate matters, signs and symptoms of certain injuries may take several hours or possibly days to show up. The injured person may seem fine shortly after the injury or while in the emergency department, but things can change.

The following stories will give you examples of what I mean and will also give the signs and symptoms of head and abdominal injuries . . . injuries that can become real killers.

*Bicycle helmets reduce the risk of a serious head injury by 80%.
Only 25 % of children ages five to fourteen-years-old wear helmets when riding.*

HEAD INJURIES

The first story is almost unbelievable because this guy should have died. The second story is a classic example of how a seemingly minor head injury turns fatal.

Believe it or Not

In 1848 Phineas Gage was working for the Rutland & Burlington railroad. While at work, an explosion hurled a three foot seven inch

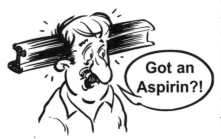

long and over one and a quarter inch diameter crowbar at him. The bar entered his left cheek and exited through the top of his head flying another 25 yards before stopping! To everyone's surprise, including Phineas, he was not dead. Some reports said he didn't even lose consciousness. He was operated on, recovered, and even returned to work but his co-workers were not happy with him. Apparently his injury caused a personality change which made him very grumpy, miserable and profane. He was let go and ended up doing some odd jobs including appearing in Barnum's museum in New York.

This is a rare case because most people who sustain an automatic lobotomy like Phineas are dead before they hit the ground. But in some cases, less serious head injuries can be fatal.

The following example demonstrates how sneaky serious head injuries can be.

He didn't seem to be hurt

Our ambulance was called at 6:30 am on a Monday morning because a lady couldn't wake her son to go to work. When we arrived he was unconscious on his bed. The history was sketchy but we did rule out a diabetic reaction or narcotics overdose. While questioning his mom about some bruises and scratches on his face, she told us he had been in a fight eight days earlier, wasn't seriously injured, and did not seek medical aid.

He was in very serious condition and not responding to anything. Further questioning revealed that a few days after the fight, his personality started to change as he became short tempered and very irritable. Questioning the mother about the events from the night before revealed that he lay on the couch, appeared very sleepy and slept for most of the evening. She told him to go to bed, which he did, and was discovered next morning unconscious. The mother then called paramedics.

We rushed him to the hospital where he died several hours later.

Head injuries are the leading cause of death due to trauma. Trauma results when violence is inflicted on the body and can be from a motor vehicle collision, a fall, or a baseball bat. Most people think that the signs and symptoms of a head injury will always show up immediately following the injury. In many cases that's true but if the signs and symptoms don't show up immediately there may be delayed effects.

Take proper care to protect your head. If you think your head is as hard as a rock, think again . . . it isn't. Here are a few tips to help you protect your head.

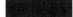

Wear the proper head protection

If you're riding a bicycle, motorcycle, skateboard, playing hockey or any other activity where a head injury is possible, make sure you wear the appropriate headgear. Wearing a bicycle helmet while riding on a snowmobile or motorcycle is not acceptable because they have different designs and will not protect your head appropriately.

Make sure the helmet you are wearing is approved by a reliable organization.

A college motorcycle instructor was test-driving a bike in front of his class in the college parking lot. He skidded on some gravel and went flying over the handlebars landing on his head. He died next day. He left a wife and two small children ages two and three.

Bicycle helmets should have an approval label from CPSC (Consumer Product Safety Commission) or Snell in the USA while in Canada it should have a CSA label (Canadian Standards Association) or Snell label.

Wearing your helmet is a great way to encourage your kids to wear theirs. You will lose credibility if you tell your kids to wear a helmet and not wear one yourself. The old line "do as I say and not as I do" is not a good way to teach safety.

I saw a man, about 35-years-old, riding his bicycle with his two kids following on their own shiny bicycles. One child was a boy about eight and the other was a girl around six. Dad was setting a good example by wearing his helmet but the kids did not have helmets on their heads. The father thought his head was important enough to protect but his children's were not.

Thinking this was wrong and not being afraid to speak up, I mentioned this to him. I don't think he was impressed, but he knew I was right.

Because head injuries are very common and can be serious, I've listed some of the signs and symptoms that may occur after a blow to the head. This is not a complete list so I strongly recommend that everyone take a recognized first aid course to learn more about head injuries and how to treat them.

Pain

There may or may not be any pain in the event of a head injury. A head injury can mask or hide other injuries. In fact, people who have a head injury may have other serious injuries like broken arms or legs and not realize it. A head injury can prevent pain perception.

Decreased level of consciousness

This is very important! When a person has sustained a head injury you may see their level of consciousness change. This means they may go from being awake and alert to confused, sleepy and comatose. They may not know the time, where they are or who they are. Ask them! This is what happened to the teenager in the above story. Blood vessels in and around the brain were bleeding and putting pressure on the brain and it took over a week for the pressure to raise enough to kill him. With other cases it could take only minutes. A person with a suspected head injury needs to get to a hospital quickly! Call an ambulance.

Combativeness

A person with a head injury can also become agitated, aggressive, and combative. In some cases, people who have been drinking may have received a head injury from an assault, fall or motor vehicle collision. Some people, after drinking alcohol and receiving a blow to the head have become aggressive with the police. There are documented cases where the police, thinking inebriation was responsible for their aggressive behavior, had thrown them in the drunk tank and left them for hours. Some have died because, once again, the blood vessels bled enough to put pressure on the brain.

Blood or straw colored fluid coming from the inside of the ears.

This could be a sign of a skull fracture. The straw colored fluid is cerebral spinal fluid and belongs in an area around your brain and spinal cord. You should be very concerned if you see this.

Poor memory

After a person has been hit on the head they may have poor memory and may repeatedly ask the same question like "what happened?"

Seizures

In some cases a person may have a seizure or convulsion immediately after an injury or days or weeks after the injury. A seizure can be a very serious medical emergency. Get help! If you do witness a seizure, call or send someone for help, protect the person by moving obstacles away from them and DO NOT attempt to insert anything into their mouth. They will not bite off their tongue.

A construction worker was accidentally tapped in the head with a nail gun. The three-inch nailed was buried in his skull. The man who was hit, but fully conscious, looked at his friend and said, "you've just nailed me in the head!" Doctors suspected he would never be able to walk or talk again. They were wrong. Six days later he walked out of the hospital under his own power. He did report, since the injury, that he had changed. "I used to like my eggs over easy, but now I like them sunny side up," he said.

Perhaps one of the old wives tales that can lead to personal injury relates to the incorrect belief that patients can swallow their tongue. A 14-year-old boy was watching television in the living room with his father. Suddenly, he stared straight ahead, clenched his fists and flopped over on to the rug. According to a younger brother who also witnessed the seizure, he then began shaking his limbs and frothing at the mouth. The father, known for his violent tendencies and who possessed no medical training, immediately picked his son up and ran to the bathroom where his wife had been relaxing in the bath. He yanked her out of the bath and threw his son in to the water, at the same time grabbing a hairbrush and attempting to ram it into the boys tightly clenched jaw. Shortly after that, the boy awoke to find himself thoroughly drenched with numerous lacerations around his mouth that required suturing. Further investigation revealed that the boy had a history of epilepsy but hadn't seized with his father present before . . . probably a good thing as he may have been fatally injured! By the time paramedics arrived, the boy was alert to time, place and person. The paramedics wheeled him on their stretcher to the ambulance while the father swore and screamed at the paramedics to hurry up, though the boy was in no immediate danger. Police had to be called when the father began beating the side of the ambulance and threatening to harm the EMS personnel. (D.L.)

Should you come across a patient who is seizing, simply protect them from hurting themselves by loosening any restrictive clothing and removing obstacles in their path. Do not attempt to introduce anything into a patient's mouth who is actively seizing. Have someone call an ambulance or call one yourself and note what areas of the body shake and for how long.

If You Suspect a Head Injury, Seek Medical Aid

Why wear a hard hat?

The following is an excerpt from one of my talks I give about injury prevention. A couple of years ago I was visiting a friend of mine. His 18 year-old son, who recently got his first full-time job on a construction site, was complaining that he had to wear a hard hat at work. "It's too awkward," he said. "It's too hot, I get too sweaty with it, and it's really uncomfortable." I responded: "Wait a minute, Shaun. I'm going to tell you why they make you wear a hard hat. You might be the safest worker in the country, but there's a guy on the second floor of this construction site who isn't as safe as you and he lets a hammer fall. Now, if this hammer hits you in the head and you're wearing a hard hat, well, it can still hurt you and you're going to know about it, but chances are you're probably not going to be that seriously injured. But if you're not wearing a hard hat, here's what is going to happen. It's going to hit your skull and it's going to fracture your skull and that's the least of your concerns, because it's also going to rupture the blood vessels that go around your brain. It can also rupture blood vessels that are actually in your brain. These blood vessels are going to bleed under quite high pressure, so you're going to end up getting a puddle of blood in and around your brain. This puddle is going to get bigger and bigger. Something has to give, and because your skull is hard it isn't going to give. But, because your brain is soft and mushy, it is going to give. If you're lucky, they get you to a big hospital where a neurosurgeon can go inside and relieve that pressure.

Now you have a brain injury, so you're going to end up in a brain injury ward where you might be for several months. Then you're going to get transferred to a place similar to a nursing home where you'll be in a wheelchair - actually, you're going to be tied to this wheelchair wheelchair because you don't have muscle control anymore. And the minute they undo these straps that hold you into the wheelchair, you're going to go face first onto the tile floor and there's not a darn thing you're going to be able to do about it.

But there's this nurse who is just a couple of years older. She's very, very attractive and a lot of fun to be around. She makes you laugh and helps you back into the wheelchair. And you think to yourself, 'Boy, I'd really like to ask you out,' but let's be serious Shaun. She's not going to date a guy who's in a wheelchair, can't remember his name half the time and has to wear diapers. She's not going to date you - get over it. You'll never be more than just friends with her. But because she's so nice to you, she gives you the best seat in the house and wheels you to the front picture window where you can watch the cars go up and down the street. In fact, you see a carload of your friends go by. Actually, they would be your ex-friends now because they have stopped visiting you several months ago and you're angry at them for it.

"Now it's dinner time, and someone wheels you to the table. They put a bib on you - you have to wear a bib now because you can't feed yourself properly. Food just falls all over in front of you and this nurse you don't really like, she's going to feed you now because the nurse that you do like is going off to a party because it's Friday night. And that hurts. So now it's bedtime. Someone wheels you back into your room that you share with three other people and helps you get into bed. After being tucked in, you lie there and you start thinking. Then you start doing what you do every other night. You lie there and you start crying, and you cry yourself to sleep as you do every night. But just before you go to sleep, one thought goes through your head, the same thought that goes through your head every night just before you fall asleep. As you lie there you think, 'My God, I have another 50 years of this.' That's why you wear a hard hat, Shaun.

ABDOMINAL INJURIES

A 31-year-old lady was taking a motorcycle safety course and during the course fell off the motorcycle. She didn't appear to be injured as she picked up the bike and continued on. At home later that evening she complained of a slight pain in the abdominal area but didn't think much about it. Later that night she showed signs of a serious injury and was taken to the hospital where she later died. She had bled to death because of a ruptured spleen.

Abdominal injuries, like head injuries, can be very sneaky or subtle. In many cases people have received injuries to their abdomen because of a fall, motor vehicle collision, or a blow (whether intentional or unintentional). The patient usually doesn't think the injury is serious. In these rare cases, sometimes an injured person has gone home and died as the lady in the story did. If the injured person, or the people around them, had understood the seriousness of the injuries perhaps the outcome could have been different.

There are two abdominal injury classifications;

Open:

An open abdominal injury occurs when the skin breaks which can be caused by stab wounds. The wound on the outside may be small, but the damage inside may be serious if organs are injured. Intestines may be exposed if the wound is large enough. Ich!

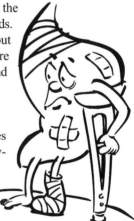

Closed:

A closed abdominal injury – the skin does not break but damage is done to the underlying organs. A kick to the abdomen can easily cause this type of injury.

If the hollow organs, such as the stomach or intestines are ruptured, the contents may spill out into the abdominal cavity and cause horrible infections. If the solid organs, such as the liver and spleen are damaged, severe internal bleeding may result.

An abdominal injury doesn't have to be an open injury to be serious. If you see a gaping wound, it may look more serious than a closed injury but this may not be the case. Often, it is the closed injuries that can sneak up and kill.

The following are some of the signs and symptoms that may be present in the event of an abdominal injury.

Pain

The person may or may not complain of pain. If there is pain, the person may lie very still because movement hurts. The person may lie in the (curled up in a ball) fetal position because this puts less pressure on the abdominal area and muscles.

Shock may be present

Because of internal bleeding, people can go into hypovolemic (due to loss of excess amounts of blood) shock. This means their blood pressure is low due to bleeding. Shock is a life-threatening condition and is irreversible if left for too long.

Bruising

This is very important. A bruise may take several hours to form after a blow and can mean the patient is bleeding internally. Seek medical aid immediately.

Distention

In some cases the abdomen may look distended — one side may look larger than the other. This could be a sign of massive internal bleeding and the blood is pooling inside the abdominal cavity. People can easily have a quart or liter of blood sloshing around their abdominal cavity and not realize it.

Abdominal injuries are the third leading cause of death due to trauma. As was pointed out in the earlier stories, an abdominal injury may not appear to be serious at first but if you suspect an abdominal injury, seek medical aid immediately.

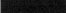

A bus lost control and crashed into a chain link fence. One of the passengers, a 40-year-old pipe fitter, was skewered through his abdomen and fastened to his seat. He said he felt like he was harpooned. Luckily the pipe missed his vital organs. Later, as doctors handed a piece of the pipe to him as a souvenir, the pipe fitter looked at the docs and with a trained eye exclaimed "inch and a quarter."

Chapter

8

STATISTICS

We often read about statistics and tend to look at them as numbers. In my line of work, emergency personnel tend to view statistics a bit differently than most people. The following story is from a call I attended and wished I hadn't. It made me look at statistics in a different light.

At 9 p.m. on December 10, 1988, our ambulance responded to a motor vehicle collision. When we arrived, we found we didn't need the jaws of life to gain access to the injured because the right side of the car was torn open. An eight-year-old boy was lying on top of his 35-year-old dad. Both of them were on the floor in the back seat, the seatbelts were stretched to their limit but somehow, in a strange manner, still attached to their bodies. The boy's torso was turned at an impossible angle so the front of his pelvis was facing in the same direction as his back.

There was no pulse; the boy was dead. I pulled him out and placed him in the ditch and thought to myself, "This shouldn't happen to a little kid." I checked the dad for signs of life but there were none. There was nothing we could do. Fifteen minutes later we went back to the fire hall.

Several days later, a police officer who had worked on the case told me more. Several hours after the crash, the police went to the small apartment where the man and his son lived to deliver the news to the wife. The woman couldn't speak English so the police had to find someone to translate. Two hours passed before the translator arrived.

You could see the fear in the woman's face because she didn't have to be told, in her native tongue, that something was terribly wrong. She took the news very hard. Who wouldn't? The police learned that the family had arrived from Poland several months earlier and that the bereaved woman didn't know a soul in the city. Her husband and only child were dead, and she was alone.

I read about this incident in the newspaper. Toxicology tests revealed that the man's blood alcohol had been four times over the legal limit. I couldn't help but think about the horror the boy felt right before the crash. Fortunately, he died quickly.

Try to put yourself in the mother's shoes. The people you love the most are dead, and here you are — not knowing a soul, not being able to speak the language, having no money to pay for a funeral and being totally alone at Christmas.

For most of us, the statistics about the people who die each year because of drinking and driving are just that — numbers printed on a sheet of paper. Sometimes we read the stories about these numbers in the newspaper. The father and son I tried to help instantly went from living, breathing human beings to numbers; statistics. For the poor woman who was left behind, her husband and child were more than numbers.

There are statistics about people who are injured or killed at their workplaces every year. We see the stories on television, hear them on the radio or read about them in newspapers. We look at the numbers but seldom give them a second thought unless we knew the people involved.

If you have ever had to break the news to the spouse of a co-worker who has been killed, you know what follows. You realize statistics refer to husbands, wives, mothers, fathers, friends, colleagues and just plain good people. It's important for us to realize the extreme mental and physical suffering that can result from an unintentional death. And think . . . almost all were preventable.

What does a person think before they die? What do they think about during weeks or months of pain spent in the burn unit due to their carelessness. Perhaps they think of the future plans made with their families. It must be awful to know you are dying and will not be able to hold your kids one last time due to the bandages and pain. What goes through your mind when you're not able to tell your spouse and kids you love them because of the tubes in your windpipe that allow you to breathe but not speak.

You must think about how and why this happened. You weren't wearing flame resistant clothing. Maybe you decided to take a silly risk doing something you've done a thousand times before. You never dreamed you would die in this manner. Unfortunately you can't reverse time and undo the mistake.

When you die, you simply become another number with all the others who died at work, in a motor vehicle collision, fall, house fire or after being hit by a drunk driver. We read the statistics but don't give them a second thought. If we don't know the people involved, these are just numbers, not actual people. Don't try telling that to their families.

9

USE THE PROPER TOOL AND SAFETY EQUIPMENT FOR THE JOB!

I think we have all done it. We try to use a four foot ladder for a job where we needed a six foot ladder. We try to use a saw that is wrong for the job. We don't have safety goggles to use with the saw so we just squint, and hope for the best. We don't have a set of safety stands that will keep the vehicle up just in case the jack slips. But that doesn't matter, the jack won't slip while I'm underneath the car, or I hope it won't.

Hardware stores are great resources. Go into them and look at the different safety devices. Talk to a salesperson and explain to them what you are trying to do. They may know of some tools or safety devices that can make the job much easier and safer.

Sometimes a person is much better off hiring someone for the job. For example, falling trees takes skill. Many professional loggers are seriously injured or killed every year while falling trees. Even though they have the training, skill and proper tools, things can go wrong. Now take a person who has no training or skill. In fact they may have never even seen a tree cut down. They go to the rental shop and rent a chainsaw. They go home and, without a clue, then attempt to cut down the thirty foot tree in their front yard. Serious injury can result and if it doesn't, there is a good chance they dropped the tree on their neighbors house or even their own. Some people may be scared to death of heights but they will get a twenty foot ladder and attempt to wash the outside windows. Their knees are shaking like a sewing machine and they are too busy worrying about falling so they don't even do a good job on the windows.

Countless people have been injured when they attempted to do a job they had no experience with or they did not use the appropriate safety tools or personal protective equipment. Don't let this happen to you. Never be afraid to seek out good advice. Take a trip to the hardware to get yourself protective gloves, goggles, a hardhat and other safety equipment you may need. Keep them around the house and never be afraid to use them.

Chapter

10

BE PREPARED FOR AN EMERGENCY

I worked as a paramedic in a town of about five thousand people. At the busiest intersection there was a low speed motor vehicle collision that caused minimal damage. One of the drivers walked over to see if the other driver was okay. The other driver was a lady about thirty years old who hadn't been wearing a seatbelt; her head hit the corner post and she received a small cut on her forehead. She had about twenty drops of blood running down her face which made the injury look much worse than it actually was. Unfortunately, for the other driver, he could not stand the sight of blood and he fainted. There were no less than seven bystanders watching him but it was about four minutes before an ambulance was called. Everyone present agreed this would be a good thing to do so someone ran to the pay phone and made the call. (This was before cell phones.) A few minutes later ambulance sirens could be heard in the distance. No one attempted to help this person. After all the ambulance was coming — the EMTs or paramedics would take care of things. When the ambulance arrived, the emergency medical technicians (EMTs) went to work. It was too late. He died. His tongue had relaxed, as it does during unconsciousness, and blocked his airway preventing him from breathing. He left a young wife and two small children behind. This shouldn't have happened.

In Japan a man was choking on a rice cake. Family members tried to remove the rice with their fingers but were unsuccessful. Things did not look good for the man until his 46-year-old daughter grabbed the vacuum cleaner, put the switch on high and stuck the hose into his mouth. It managed to suck out the obstruction and the man was fully recovered before the ambulance arrived.

I don't know if the people who witnessed this tragedy had any first aid skills or if they were too afraid to help. Either way, the man died and he didn't have to. All someone had to do was open his airway and he, most likely, would have started breathing on his own. This would have been a simple faint instead of a fatality but no one was prepared for this emergency.

If emergencies happened only when you expected and were prepared for them they wouldn't be emergencies. Unfortunately, an emergency can happen to anyone, at any time, and in any place. You have to be ready for them. You have to be trained and prepared!

Ask yourself the following questions:

- If someone in your family started to choke at dinner, do you know how to administer abdominal thrusts to clear the airway?

- Do you know how to shut off the power in your house when a flood occurs?

- In the event of a fire in your home; do you have an escape plan?

- When was the last time you checked your smoke detectors to see if they really work? When was the last time you practiced a fire drill with your children? Have you ever?

- If a blizzard or ice storm occurred and your power went out for three days, how would you handle it? (Remember, this means no heat, lights, stove, and heaven forbid, television!) While writing this book, Buffalo, New York received over six feet of snow in a blizzard.

- If a tornado warning is issued, do you know what to do? Do you know how to protect your family?

These are just a few examples of emergencies that can happen. The following are a few suggestions to help you deal with emergencies.

- Take a first aid course from a recognized agency. Everyone in your family should take one.

- Keep a disaster supply kit handy and well stocked. You may never need it but if you do, you will be relieved you took the time to put one together. The following are some of the items that should be in a disaster kit:

- A water supply to last a minimum three days (one gallon of water per person, per day). Your hot water tank holds approximately 40 gallons (160 litres) of water and a toilet tank holds about four gallons (16 litres). If you live in an area prone to flooding, consider including water purification tablets in your kit. Flooding can contaminate municipal water supplies.

- Food to last a family for three or more days. (Most homes will have enough unless there are teenagers in the home.) If your power is disrupted the food in your freezer should keep for three days if the door is kept closed. Canned food stores well and remember to put a manual can opener in the kit. Store food staples in heavy duty plastic containers and take into consideration family members special diets (for example diabetes or allergies).

- One sleeping bag or heavy blanket for each person. If you live in an area like Winnipeg, Manitoba or Fairbanks, Alaska, a blanket just won't be warm enough if the power is out for any length of time.

- A first aid kit and supply of medications for anyone in the family who needs them.

- Extra clothing for each person.

- A portable radio (AM/FM) in good working condition, with spare batteries. Make sure the batteries are the proper size.

- At least one flashlight with spare (appropriate size) batteries.

- A fire extinguisher.

As you can see, most homes will have many of the items listed. It's just a matter of keeping them together and available.

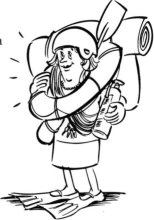

- If traveling in the winter, keep a supply of winter clothes including warm boots, a parka, winter hat and mitts in your vehicle. Make sure you have enough for each person traveling. Also keep a sleeping bag, shovel and some emergency food such as chocolate bars in the car. If you are stuck, run your vehicle for five to ten minutes at a time so the heater can warm up your vehicle. For this reason it's important to travel with a full tank of gas. Keep a window opened a few inches to help prevent carbon monoxide poisoning and make sure your exhaust pipe is clear of snow. In a blizzard you may have to check for this on a regular basis because snow can blow in fast and cover your exhaust.

- Many people believe a candle will keep them warm in a car. Think about this, it's minus 30 degrees; you are surrounded by three tons of steel and glass. Do you really think a candle alone will keep you warm? Not likely. Be prepared. You will need lots of warm clothes.

Chapter

11

FIRE SAFETY

We were called to a house trailer fire with the ambulance. When we arrived the trailer was fully engulfed in flames. The firefighters quickly put the fire out but it was too late. Two adults died in their beds from carbon monoxide posioning while they slept. They never knew what happened.

The children weren't so lucky. All four of the children ranging from ages two to nine years were found at the back door. They were burned beyond recognition. They tried to get out but couldn't. The door had been latched closed and it was too high for them to reach. They died a horrible death. The fear and pain those poor kids went through is unimaginable.

I've attended numerous scenes where people have died or have been seriously burned from fires in their homes. No one expects a fire. Everyone thinks it will never happen to them. Fires always happen to someone else. People think they are immune to a fire happening in their home. Fires are scary and most people do not realize what happens in a fire and how scary and dangerous they are . . . unless you have been through the horror of a fire.

A fire in your home is not like what you see on television

The fire started off small. It was caused by a hot ash that had been knocked off the end of a cigarette. It fell between the cushions and smoldered for hours. At 3:00 am it finally burst into a small flame that gradually grew producing heat and smoke. You took the battery out of your smoke detector two weeks ago because the low battery alarm was beeping and it was irritating you — **it didn't go off.** You and your family are upstairs sleeping unaware that the small fire is growing quickly producing heat and poisonous smoke. Finally the couch bursts into flames and quickly spreads to the drapes. In fewer than one and a half minutes, the living room and entire lower floor are full of thick, black poisonous smoke. This heat and smoke is quietly making its way up the stairs to the bedrooms. Escaping the house through the lower floors is now impossible. The temperature is 600 degrees F (315 degrees C) and the smoke is so thick you can't see your hand in front of your face.

Suddenly your kids run into your bedroom screaming. You wake up and it takes a few seconds for you to realize what is happening. The thick, black choking smoke and heat is filling your bedroom. You hug your children as the heat and smoke fill your lungs. Your children are screaming. You pick them up and try to run down the stairs to safety. It's too hot and the smoke is too thick; this can't be happening! We're going to die! You feel yourself going unconscious. Just before you die, you wake up from the nightmare. You go to your children's bedroom, look at them and smile. Then, you go downstairs and replace the battery in the smoke detector. Something you should have done weeks ago.

In England, a dog bit through an aerosol can of hairspray. The spray that streamed out was ignited by a gas fireplace. The aerosol can acted like a blowtorch. The fire caused a lot of damage and also killed two cats that lived there.

Unfortunately the first story in this chapter was not a dream. Real children died and it didn't have to happen. The following is safety information to help you make your homes safer. I strongly recommend you seek out and read further information on fire safety. Your local fire department is a good place to start gathering further information.

Smoke detectors

You've probably heard the expression "smoke detectors save lives." It's true, they do. But do you really understand how they save lives. It's simple. They buy you time; time to escape; time to save your life.

In many cases people have smoke detectors in their home that don't work. The battery could be dead or the smoke detector hasn't been cleaned or it's been painted over. A smoke detector that doesn't work is useless. Worse than that, if you think it's functioning, it gives you a false sense of security.

Close to 90% of residential fire deaths occur in homes without smoke alarms or in homes where the smoke alarms are not functioning.

Many home fires happen at night when people are asleep. Smoke alarms should be placed outside sleeping areas. Install one in every major area of the house, including the laundry room. Test smoke alarms regularly. When an alarm gives a low battery signal (often a beep every 30 – 60 seconds) replace the battery promptly.

We attended a call at 4 a.m. for a fire in a condominium. As soon as the firefighters entered the building they found a seventeen-year-old male a few feet from the door. He was not breathing and did not have a pulse. We treated the teen without success and he was pronounced dead in the hospital shortly after.

In this case the teen had come home after a party. He started to cook a snack and fell asleep on the couch. A fire started in the pot and spread to the cupboards. By the time he woke up, the room was filled with smoke. He tried to make it to the front door that was less than five feet away. He didn't make it. The batteries from the smoke detector were taken out two weeks earlier because the low battery alarm had been going off. There was less than $5000 damage to the kitchen but the human cost was immeasurable.

Here's a few tips about smoke detectors.

- Be sure everyone in the household is familiar with the sound of the smoke detector and understands that it means **GET OUT NOW!**

- Here's one way to test an alarm: light a candle and then put it out. Let the smoke from the candle drift into the alarm. Do this at least once a month. Some models have a test button you can press to sound the alarm. Note that this test may be useful for testing the alarm itself, but it may not test the smoke sensing system. Follow the manufacturer's directions for testing your particular smoke detector. You can purchase smokeless aerosol spray for testing smoke detectors. You just spray the contents at the detector and it will imitate the effects of smoke. Always follow the directions on the can.

- Clean the detector on a regular basis. Dust build-up can cause false alarms or malfunctions. Follow the manufacturer's directions for cleaning.

- If you have been away for a few days, check your detectors when you return. The low battery alarm may have been going off when you were away and the battery is now completely dead.

One of my friends, who will remain nameless, had just started a new job as a fire prevention officer. He was doing a house inspection and was using the artificial smoke spray to test smoke detectors in a lady's house. As he was checking the detector in the living room he noticed it wasn't activating. He sprayed the detector several times but it still wouldn't go off. He explained to the lady that she should have it replaced. She politely told him he was testing her doorbell chime.

Have an Escape Plan

Very few families actually have an escape plan in case of a fire; even fewer have practiced their plan. Your kids have fire drills on a regular basis in school. You should have a plan at home not only for your sake but also for your children's sake. After all, your children have a much higher chance of dying in a fire in your home than they do at school.

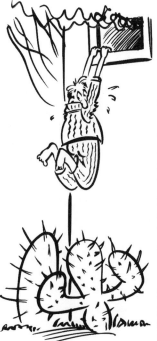

Once you are aware there's a fire in your home, you must get out immediately. An escape plan helps you do this. Draw a house plan and mark escape routes from every location. Determine a primary and alternative escape route from each room and then decide on a place where everyone is to meet as soon as they're out of the house. This could be a tree, a street light or a neighbor's front door but make sure the meeting place is a safe distance from the house. Practice your escape plan regularly. Have someone sound the alarm, then rehearse what you would do and where you would go in case of a fire.

Review the plan frequently with all family members. Ask your local fire department for more fire prevention information. They will be happy to give you information and answer any questions.

Tell your children if there's a fire they must not hide. This makes it much more difficult for the firefighters to find them. Explain to them that if they see a firefighter during a fire he will be wearing a mask and will look scary; explain that they should run *to* them Also tell your children that when there's a fire, it's okay to break a window to call for help.

If there's a fire in your home, the following are good responses:

A 20-year-old man was camping with his friends. They decided to fill a bottle with gasoline and throw it into a fire. When it exploded a large piece of glass flew into one of the campers' neck. He was flown by helicopter to the hospital at around two am. He is expected to survive.

- If you've been sleeping, get out of bed and crawl to the door on the floor. Smoke and heat rise so it's cooler and easier to breathe on the floor.

- Touch the door. If it's warm, don't open it. If the door is cool to touch, open it very slowly because there may be intense heat on the other side. If the hallway is full of smoke or if you can see fire, close the door and use an alternative route out. I have a phone in my room and I put my cordless phone in my little girls' room. This way they could call 9-1-1 if they couldn't get out of our condominium.

Close the door.

When leaving the building, stay low and close the doors behind you. Closed doors will help slow the spread of fire. Smoke and heat from a fire can fill a house in a very short time. Closing the door to the room where the fire is can slow the spread of fire to the rest of the home. Most doors in public buildings have fire rated doors. This means it will take a fire so many minutes to burn through. It may be 30 minutes or more. In the event of a fire many buildings are designed so that the doors will close automatically in the event of a fire. This helps to slow the spread of the fire.

The doors in your home are probably not fire rated but if closed, may help slow the spread of the fire and poisonous smoke.

- Get out of the building and stay out. No one should go back in side until the fire department tells you it's safe to do so.

One man escaped his house during a fire. When he was safely out he realized his pet dog was still in. He ran back into the house to search for him. By the time the firefighters found him, he was dead.

- Once you're out of the burning building, go to the designated meeting spot and make sure everyone is accounted for.

- Phone the fire department from a neighbor's house. You want to exit the burning house as soon as possible.

- If you can't get out of the house because of the smoke and heat, close the door of the room you're in. Plug any cracks under the door with bedding to prevent smoke from entering. Open a window and exit if you can. If you're on an upper floor scream for help and try to get someone's attention. Don't jump out of the window unless there isn't another choice.

This young man was very lucky. He was asleep in his bedroom when the smoke detector went off. The smoke was very thick and filled the rooms in his apartment. The rooms were completely filled from the ceiling to about three feet off the floor so he crawled and made it to safety. The reason for the delayed alarm activation is that he had taken it down to replace the battery. He then placed it on the kitchen counter instead of replacing it on the ceiling. The alarm didn't go off until the smoke level had dropped low enough to reach the kitchen counter.

Alcohol contributes to 40% of residential fire deaths. Alcohol use is involved in about 25%-50% of adolescent and adult deaths associated with water.

Chimney Fires

During Christmas holidays, we responded to several chimney fires. They became quite a hassle for the people who lived in the houses.

Imagine that you're sitting on a bearskin rug in front of a fireplace; enjoying a glass of wine with someone you love. What could be more romantic? It's a scene right out of a picture book.

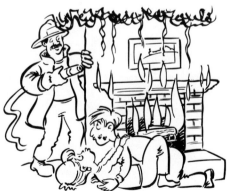

Then, all of a sudden, your fire begins to roar, and the neighbors are amazed to see flames and sparks flying out your chimney. It looks like a volcano. Next, you have to face the embarrassment of having a bunch of firefighters march into your house, making a terrible mess. A truly frightening experience, and not exactly the kind of evening you had in mind.

A slow-burning fire might seem preferable because it's less obvious. But it can produce high enough temperatures to damage the chimney structure.

Chimney fires occur when chimneys are not kept clean. A by-product of combustion is a residue called creosote. Creosote sticks to the inside of the chimney, and if it catches fire, it burns with great intensity.

Here are a few tips to help ensure that when you use a wood burning stove or fireplace, the fire will remain in the right place and not race up the chimney:

- Have the chimney inspected and cleaned on a regular basis by a certified chimney sweep.

- Use dry, seasoned woods only. Having dry wood is more important than the variety of wood you burn.

- Build smaller, hotter fires that burn more completely and produce less smoke.

- Don't use your fireplace or wood-burning stove to burn card board, wrapping paper, trash or Christmas trees. Burning these substances can spark a chimney fire.

- If you use a wood stove, install stovepipe thermometers to help monitor flue temperatures.

We attended a chimney fire once when the owner of the house had tried to burn his Christmas tree in the fireplace. The interesting part is the tree was artificial. He was very determined and put enough wood, cardboard and whatever else he could find around the house to burn the tree! The tree was flame retardant but not fire proof.

A month before Christmas our fire trucks responded to a house at three a.m. The deck and the whole back of the house were on fire. For-

tunately, the man and his two young daughters escaped without injuries. Earlier that night the occupants had a fire in the fireplace. Thinking all the ashes were cool, they put the ashes in a large plastic garbage bag and placed it on the deck. Unfortunately, the coals were not as cold as they thought and smoldered for hours eventually bursting into flames which spread to the house.

We were familiar with the house. Two weeks earlier the mother had died of cancer. Fire doesn't doesn't show mercy.

A final note about fires

Even a small fire in your home is going to leave one heck of a mess. Imagine four or five firefighters with dirty boots knocking over furniture and spraying your house with gallons of water. There will be dirt, soot, ash and holes chopped into walls and ceilings and since most of the firefighters are guys, we won't clean up after ourselves. You'll be stuck with the mess!

Don't let a fire happen in your home!

12

SAFETY IS NOT ONLY ABOUT LIFE AND DEATH

So often in safety education we hear "if you take risks, you could be killed." That's true, but there is more to it. The quality of life after an injury isn't discussed. I've been involved in some situations where the people who have been injured wished they had died. I remember one person who told me, over and over again, he wished he was dead after breaking his neck and becoming completely paralyzed. These are pretty powerful words . . . especially when I knew he meant it. He lived in a hospital bed for another four years before his wish came true

Sometimes in the safety profession I think we put all the focus on life and death. We say, "if you take risks you could get killed. If you don't wear your seatbelt, you could die." That's true but I think we forget about the importance of the quality of life after an injury. There are many injuries that can be devastating. The pain and suffering from some injuries are incomprehensible. I've never been seriously injured and don't want to be but if I received the injuries some people I treated had received, I'm not sure I would want to continue living. I guess a person really doesn't know until they are in that situation.

I know some people who have been horribly injured and have done amazing things with the remaining years of their lives and others who have wanted to end their lives.

The next time you consider taking a risk, don't think only about being killed . . . think about the quality of life that you would have if things go wrong.

13

IT'S NOT THE FALL THAT KILLS YOU; IT'S THE SUDDEN STOP

We responded to a drinking establishment where a 56-year-old man tripped and fell face first down four stairs. He landed on his face with enough force to hyperextend his neck (force his head violently backward). His neck was broken causing his spinal cord to be severely damaged. He was completely paralyzed from the neck down and was on a respirator for the remaining four and a half years of his life. This happened because of a fall down four small steps.

A college professor received near fatal head injuries when he fell off his roof onto the driveway. At the time he was shoveling the snow from the roof and fell headfirst.

In the USA during 1999, 15,447 people died as a result of falls. 1,295 of those died from a fall on or from stairs or steps. That's a lot of people. Falls are one of the most common causes of unintentional death and they happen to people of all ages. Falls not only kill people, they cause severe injuries that can affect the person for as long as they live.

You can die or be seriously injured from many different kinds of injuries because of a fall. The fall can be from something as low as a chair or as high as a roof. Both can be deadly. The following are some of the injuries that can happen to you because of a fall.

Landing On Your Head

Landing on your head is especially dangerous and it doesn't have to be from a high height to cause major damage. If you fall and your head hits first, your skull is going to receive a lot of force. The force will be transmitted to your brain. Blood vessels in and around your brain can rupture causing them to bleed. Since the blood won't be able to leak out of your skull, pressure will build up in the brain. Landing on your head also increases the risk of spinal cord damage.

Police officers responded to a 61-year-old possible suicide. Police believed the woman was going to jump from the 6th floor ledge of her apartment building. Police later discovered she was just out for a smoke. This was common practice for her.

Spinal Cord Damage

Your spinal cord is about 18 inches long and starts at the brain and runs down an opening in the spine. The brain sends messages to the muscles in your body. These messages run down your spinal cord and branch off into smaller nerves. If the spinal cord is damaged, the messages from the brain don't reach the muscles they were intended for. When the messages don't reach the muscles, the muscles don't work and the person is paralyzed.

When a person lands on their head during a fall the chances of a broken neck is quite high. If the spinal cord is damaged in the neck, one of the worst injuries that can happen to a person may result. This is quadriplegia; the person is paralyzed from the neck down. This is what happened to the man in the first story of this chapter. Diving injuries can often cause quadriplegia. This happens when a person dives into a body of water that is not deep enough such as a pond, lake or pool and they hit their head on the bottom. Tremendous force is exerted on the neck and the spinal cord can be damaged. Many people are injured when they dive into back yard or hotel swimming pools. If they dive off a diving board they often hit the upslope of the pool. This is the part of the pool that slopes up from the deep end to the shallow end. Keep in mind that most backyard and hotel pools cannot safely accommodate diving.

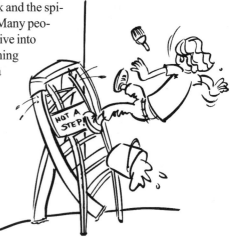

The diaphragm is a muscle sheet found near the bottom of the ribcage and enables breathing. The nerves that supply it come from high in the neck. If the nerves are damaged, you will not only lose the use of your arms and legs but the diaphragm will not work. You will most likely need a respirator to breath. You have probably seen people in this condition. They have a hole in their throat and have a tube connected to it. The tube is connected to a machine that will do breathing work by blowing air into the lungs. This is usually permanent.

An eighteen-year-old man dove off a diving board during a backyard pool party. When he surfaced he was floating face down. His friends thought he was joking and didn't do anything to help him. Several minutes passed until they finally realized something was very wrong. They carried him out of the pool onto the deck and started mouth-to-mouth resuscitation. A short while later he started to breath on his own. He is now confined to a wheelchair and paralyzed from the neck down.

Broken Bones

You are not made of rubber. When you fall, bones will break. When bones break they have sharp ends that jab into the muscles and flesh around the bones. This causes internal bleeding. For example: if you break a femur (thighbone) the muscles will contract and jab the sharp ends of the bones into your thigh causing them to bleed. Each broken femur can sometimes bleed a quart (over a litre) of blood or more. Those sharp ends can also dislodge fat into your bloodstream creating an embolism. This chunk of fat will work its way to the brain or lungs via the bloodstream and will eventually lodge somewhere. If it lodges in the brain, a stroke may result. If it lodges in the lungs, you won't be able to breath and you may die.

Internal Damage

Falling people accelerate very quickly. When they hit the ground they stop immediately. For fractions of a second, organs such as the liver and heart will continue to travel in a downward motion. This puts a lot of force on the organs and because they have tissue connecting them, the tissue stretches and may rip or tear organs resulting in severe bleeding. A person can bleed to death without seeing one drop of blood externally. These are called deceleration injuries caused from stopping too fast. These injuries can also happen when a motor vehicle hits a tree, wall or another vehicle.

A man was washing the outside windows of his house while stand-ing on a stepladder. He lost his balance and fell. Unfortunately, he landed on a picket fence and received a large a gash on his leg. Considering all things, he was quite lucky because it could have been worse.

Tips to prevent falling.

- Always, watch where you're stepping.

- Keep stairways and areas where people walk clear of objects that can be tripped over.

- Rugs and carpets should be smooth and creaseless to prevent tripping.

- Keep your steps and sidewalks free of snow and ice.

- Use appropriate length ladders for the job. Don't use a six-foot ladder for a twelve-foot job.

- At work, always follow the rules and wear your fall protection devices if needed.

- If you're uncomfortable with heights, hire someone to clean or paint the eavestrough, shovel snow from the roof, wash the out side windows or any other jobs you may find uncomfortable. The savings can be more than money.

While writing this chapter I treated a man who was building a house. He climbed a ladder onto the garage roof to nail shingles in place. The roof was about eleven feet high and as he stepped from the ladder onto the roof with his right foot, he stepped on some plastic that was sticking out from under the shingles. His foot slipped and he fell feet first onto the ground. When he landed, he heard a loud crack. When we arrived, his leg had a new bend to it. About three inches below his knee his leg was at a 90-degree angle.

LISTEN TO YOUR BODY

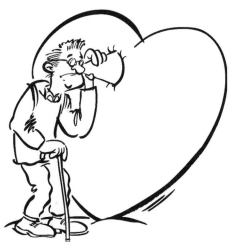

Many people will go through their entire lives without being seriously injured. This isn't so with medical emergencies. Sooner or later you stand a very good chance of suffering a heart attack, stroke or some other type of medical emergency. Hopefully your emergency won't kill you. Many of the people who die from heart attacks or strokes have had important warning signs that something very serious may be on the horizon. Some people choose to ignore the signs while others just don't realize the seriousness of the situation. Either way, the consequences are the same.

Heart Attack... It Can Happen to You

At two o'clock in the morning, January 9th, 1998 our ambulance was called to a house where a 42-year-old man needed help. We drove up to the house, took our medical kits and knocked on the front door. A beautiful little girl, about 10 years old answered the door. She had tears streaming down her cheeks. She was scared to death. She looked at us and said "It's my dad, he's upstairs." We quickly ran up the stairs. On the bedroom floor was a lady doing cardiopulmonary resuscitation. We immediately asked her to take her little girl out of the room. We didn't want her to see what was going to happen next. That morning we put needles in his arms, we put a tube down his throat so he could breathe, and we tried to shock his heart back to life. We did everything we possibly could for him. He died anyway. The sad part is this did not have to happen. He had been complaining of chest pain since 10:00 pm. So, for four hours he sat around his house having chest pain and didn't do anything to help himself. He was having a heart attack and he didn't know it, or, didn't want to believe it. He died because of his ignorance, reluctance, or stubbornness to get help. Either way, his little girl is without a father.

In New Zealand a 49-year-old man was found to have the highest level of cholesterol ever. His reading was 43 millimoles per litre. That would be 1,660 in the U.S. system. Normal levels are 5.2 and 200 in the U.S. system. Time for a diet change.

As paramedics we see situations like this time and time again. A person will have chest pain and will wait an hour, three hours, eight hours, ten hours, and then go into cardiac arrest. If you're brought into the emergency department in cardiac arrest, your chances are extremely slim of walking out of the hospital. But if you get into the hospital as soon as the chest pain starts and receive appropriate care, your chances for full recovery are very good. Presently there are drugs and medications that will dissolve blockages in heart arteries thereby restoring the required blood supply and oxygen to the heart. In order for those drugs to work, you have to get into the medical system as quickly as you possibly can. If you wait too long, the drugs won't work. When you're having a heart attack, time is crucial. Time is heart muscle.

The following isn't meant to take the place of a first aid or CPR course. I strongly recommend you take one from a recognized agency. Here are some of the signs and symptoms you may feel or see in someone who is possibly having a heart attack.

Pain – It may be described as a squeezing, heavy feeling, tightness or a burning sensation in the chest. The pain may have started without any kind of exertion. The pain may be very severe or it may be very mild and does not go away.

The pain may radiate through the arms or either shoulder or jaw. It can even radiate to the back.

Sometimes the pain may feel like indigestion. It some cases it may be hard to tell the difference between indigestion and a heart attack. Breathing deeper or shallower will not affect the pain.

Skin – The skin may be very pale and sweaty. In some cases the skin may feel cool to the touch

Shortness of breath – A person having a heart attack may complain of shortness of breath. This means they are having a hard time breathing. Sometimes, because of the damaged heart, blood and fluid can back up into the lungs. The fluid then fills the little air spaces in the lungs. This is called congestive heart failure. It can also be called pulmonary edema (fluid in the lungs)

Nausea and vomiting – A person may complain of nausea or they may vomit.

Anxiety – People may appear to be very anxious when having a heart attack and feel that death is near.

Denial – *This is important!* Many people will deny they are having a heart attack. They think they are too young, too healthy or too tough and it can't be happening to them; so they deny it. Everyone knows someone who can be very stubborn at times. In fact they might be reading this book right now.

If you deny you are having a heart attack your denial may kill you! (Or you might drown on de Nile . . . get it! Ha.)

If you or someone else experiences similar signs and symptoms, call 9-1-1. There may be a major medical problem happening before your eyes.

Quality of life – Besides killing you, the delay of medical aid in a medical emergency can have an effect on your quality of life. If you start having chest pain, recognize a problem, get into the hospital and get the appropriate treatment, within two or three weeks you could be back at home doing the things you enjoy. You're back playing with your children, or grandchildren. You're back at work doing the job you like and doing the things you enjoy.

But, if you wait, while experiencing chest pain, and delay medical treatment, you might not die. You could become a cardiac cripple. All you'll be able to do is to get up from the couch, walk to the bathroom, come back, sit and rest for the next few hours because you're exhausted. That's all the physical exertion your heart can take. I don't know about you, but I wouldn't be happy with that quality of life, especially if it was preventable.

Chapter

15

WHEN YOU SEE A DANGEROUS SITUATION, FIX IT IMMEDIATELY

Several years ago I was involved in a situation for which I have to take full responsibility. I was getting ready for a night shift at the fire hall and as I was walking out to the van I stepped on a patch of ice on the front sidewalk. My feet shot out from under me but I was able to re-cover. As I continued on to the van I thought to myself, "this is danger-ous. I've got to fix it." One thing led to another and I didn't do anything. At 2 a.m. I received a call from my neighbor, Paul, who told me my wife had fallen and broken her arm. What happened was this: my daughters were three-years-old and four-months-old when this happened. In the middle of the night the three-year-old's temperature had shot up and she was complaining of a stiff and sore neck. This is a possible sign of men-ingitis and that's something you don't want to joke around with. She had already put the infant in the car seat and as she was carrying our three-year-old to the car, she stepped on the same patch of ice I stepped on and landed on her shoulder, breaking it in three different places.

I had to take two weeks holidays to stay home and take care of everyone. For a non-domesticated male, this included cooking and clean-ing which was a huge challenge.

When I think about this incident I realize how lucky I was. What if it was my daughter's head that hit the concrete and not my ex-wife's shoul-der? I've treated people who have died or received severe brain damage after hitting their head on the concrete. This would have created a whole different ripple effect from my wife's fall and I would have been respon-sible.

How many times have you noticed a dangerous situation and just walked by as if it wasn't there? Or you were in a rush and didn't take the time to fix the dangerous situation because there were more pressing things to do. Granted, most of the time nothing will happen. No one will be injured and life will go on as usual. Unfortunately, for many people, life won't go on as usual. Because of their own negligence or someone else's, people will be hurt and many will be seriously injured.

It can be as simple as leaving your shoes or books on the stairs causing a family member to trip and fall head first breaking their neck. Or it could be something more complicated such as not turning off circuit breakers while working on electrical equipment. Two different scenarios but equally as serious.

In most cases it only takes a second or two to fix a dangerous situation. Wiping up a spill or picking up a shovel doesn't take long and it can save you or someone else from a fall that could result in an injury.

A 75-year-old man sat down on his outhouse seat. The floor and part of the wall collapsed and he fell into the five-foot hole. He spent three smelly days in the hole before a mail carrier heard his screams for help. Fortunately he didn't fall into the deepest part. "It was hard to get a breath down there," he said after being rescued. He was treated for dehydration and scratches that became infected.

When you see a dangerous situation, fix it immediately!

Chapter

16

IT'S UP TO YOU

A lot of people are responsible for their own injuries. They have no one to blame but themselves. It could be they reached too far while standing on a ladder. They knew this little move was risky but they did it anyway. Then they fell, landing on their head. Who's fault is it?

Maybe they were smoking while fueling up their lawnmower. The fumes catch fire. They receive second and third degree burns to their face, chest and arms. Who's fault is it? They knew the act was dangerous but did it anyway.

We have to take responsibility for our own actions. You are the person who has the most influence for your safety and the safety of your children before they are old enough to make decisions on their own. Take that responsibility. It's an important one.

Chapter

17

IT'S UP TO THE OTHER GUY TOO

Yes, sometimes people get hurt or killed when they are doing things in a safe manner.

Before holiday's dad makes sure the tires are inflated properly. He ensures the vehicle has a complete mechanical inspection. He is sober and has had enough sleep the night before. The kids are sitting quietly in the back seat and they aren't distracting him. Everything is fine. Then it happens. The person driving the car coming towards them is tired. He had a few too many drinks the night before. He dozes off….just for a second. Long enough to cross the center line and wipe out an entire family.

Remember, you're the other guy to everyone else. Your family is counting on you, your co-workers are counting on you and a lot of people you don't even know are counting on you not to hurt or kill them. Be responsible. It's important.

ONE MORE THING . . .

I hope you found the book interesting but more importantly, useful. The goal of this book was to get you thinking about how easily injuries can happen and how permanent they can be. It is also meant to give you some solid safety advice. Hopefully the stories and the tips will encourage you to think about safety for a long time.

I love my job as a firefighter and as a paramedic. But after twenty years attending people who have been seriously injured or died as a result of their injuries, I now realize I don't want to deal with the injuries. I would rather prevent them from happening in the first place. Prevention is less glamorous than screaming up to a house fire or motor vehicle collision in a fire truck or ambulance and treating the injured victims. It's less glamorous, but I think all firefighters and ambulance crews wish the tragedies never happened.

I would love to talk to your organization on injury prevention. If you're looking for a speaker, give me a call.

Thanks for reading and take care,
Martin Lesperance
September 2002.
www.safety-speaker.com

ABOUT THE AUTHOR

While still employed as a firefighter, Martin Lesperance leads an energetic life as a speaker, author and father and has been involved in emergency medical services for the past 20 years. During his career he has also designed safety programs for several major companies. Lesperance owns Safety Health Publishing Inc. which specializes in first aid and emergency care but also designs books, posters and tapes to help people think about safety twenty-four hours a day.

Lesperance has authored several books including *Kids for Keeps: Preventing Injuries to Children.*, *I Won't be into Work Today – Preventing Injuries at Home, Work and Play* and *What Do You Mean I'm Stressed – Recognizing And Managing Your Stress*. His reputation as an expert in safety and injury prevention has grown nationally and he has appeared on numerous television and radio programs across North America. He has also spoken to organizations including Huntsman Corporation, New Mexico Mutual Casualty Company and Los Alamos National Laboratory. His humor and extensive experience as a firefighter makes Lesperance a very popular speaker.

The father of two young girls, Lesperance enjoys hiking, kayaking, skiing and was an amateur boxing silver medalist at the 1971 Canada Winter Games. He also competed in the World Fire Fighter Games in the Toughest Fire Fighter Alive competition in 1997.

Visit his website at www.safety-speaker.com or www.safetyhealthpublishing.com

Book Lesperance To Speak At Your Safety Meeting Or Conference Now

Some of Lesperance's most popular talks include:

1. **I Won't Be Into Work Today** – Preventing Injuries At Home, Work and Play
2. **What Do You Mean I'm Stressed** – Recognizing And Managing Your Stress
3. **Medical Emergencies** – What You Should Know To Save Your Life

Visit www.safety-speaker.com

Books

What Do You Mean I'm Stressed – Recognizing And Managing Your Stress — *This 64 page book takes a fun look at stress including what causes it, how to recognize it and how to reduce it. (The book can include a customized message to your employees)*

What Do You Mean I'm Stressed and *Safety Tips That Can Save Your Butt* **are also on CD and audio tape. A great way for employees to learn about injury prevention and stress**

Safety Videos by Martin

1. **I Won't Be Into Work Today** – Preventing Injuries At Home, Work and Play
2. **Silly Little Risks** – Talking To Teens
3. **Protect Your Head** – You Only Have One
4. **Heart Attack** – It Could Happen To You.
5. **The Weekend Warriors**

To view the videos go to www.safetyvideos.ca or www.safetyhealthpublishing.com

For Free Safety Articles Visit www.safetyhealthpublishing.com Feel free to use these articles for your in-house newsletters.

For more information, call 1-888-278-8964 or (403) 225-2011